<u>Heada</u>

<u>(Easy to use Diary for Children)</u>

This Diary belongs to

....

....

This is an easy to use diary for children and teenagers.

It is convenient for all kids – they just need to check things off and add one word answers.

The size is a convenient medium size 6" X 9" and can be easily carried in a backpack whenever necessary.

It has spaces to mark the location of the headache, time started, ended, duration, other symptoms as well as plenty of space for additional notes if there are specific patterns which need to be tracked .

It has the typical suggested triggers plus spaces to note down own triggers.

Adequate spaces have been provided to write down relief measures and again more spaces for notes which are crucial.

Date:..................... Day of Week:......................

| Time Occurred | | Time Ended | |

Type of headache you have: Tick the Right one.

Sinus   Tension   Migraine   Cluster   Hypertension

Severity on a Scale of 1-10 : Tick the right number

| 1 | 2 | 3 | 4 | 5 | 6 | 7 | 8 | 9 | 10 |

Triggers: Tick the Right One

Stress, anger or sadness	Loud Noises
Missed eating a meal	Period
Slept too little or too much	Too much sun
Foods (name)	Medicine (name)

Others

How was the Headache relieved:

Medicines (name)

Sleep/ Rest

Others

Additional Notes

_____

_____

_____

Date:....................... Day of Week:.........................

Time Occurred		Time Ended	

Type of headache you have: Tick the Right one.

Sinus   Tension   Migraine   Cluster   Hypertension

Severity on a Scale of 1-10 : Tick the right number

1	2	3	4	5	6	7	8	9	10

Triggers: Tick the Right One

Stress, anger or sadness	Loud Noises
Missed eating a meal	Period
Slept too little or too much	Too much sun
Foods (name)	Medicine (name)
Others	

How was the Headache relieved:

Medicines (name)

Sleep/ Rest

Others

Additional Notes

Date:....................   Day of Week:......................

Time Occurred		Time Ended	

Type of headache you have: Tick the Right one.

Sinus   Tension   Migraine   Cluster   Hypertension

Severity on a Scale of 1-10 : Tick the right number

1	2	3	4	5	6	7	8	9	10

Triggers: Tick the Right One

Stress, anger or sadness	Loud Noises
Missed eating a meal	Period
Slept too little or too much	Too much sun
Foods (name)	Medicine (name)

Others

How was the Headache relieved:

Medicines (name)

Sleep/ Rest

Others

Additional Notes

Date:...................... Day of Week:........................

| Time Occurred | | Time Ended | |

Type of headache you have: Tick the Right one.

Sinus   Tension   Migraine   Cluster   Hypertension

Severity on a Scale of 1-10 : Tick the right number

| 1 | 2 | 3 | 4 | 5 | 6 | 7 | 8 | 9 | 10 |

Triggers: Tick the Right One

Stress, anger or sadness	Loud Noises
Missed eating a meal	Period
Slept too little or too much	Too much sun
Foods (name)	Medicine (name)

Others

How was the Headache relieved:

Medicines (name)

Sleep/ Rest

Others

Additional Notes

Date:......................   Day of Week:.......................

Time Occurred		Time Ended	

Type of headache you have: Tick the Right one.

Sinus   Tension   Migraine   Cluster   Hypertension

Severity on a Scale of 1-10 : Tick the right number

1	2	3	4	5	6	7	8	9	10

Triggers: Tick the Right One

Stress, anger or sadness	Loud Noises
Missed eating a meal	Period
Slept too little or too much	Too much sun
Foods (name)	Medicine (name)

Others

How was the Headache relieved:

Medicines (name)

Sleep/ Rest

Others

Additional Notes

Date:..................... Day of Week:.......................

Time Occurred		Time Ended	

Type of headache you have: Tick the Right one.

| Sinus | Tension | Migraine | Cluster | Hypertension |

Severity on a Scale of 1-10 : Tick the right number

1	2	3	4	5	6	7	8	9	10

Triggers: Tick the Right One

Stress, anger or sadness	Loud Noises
Missed eating a meal	Period
Slept too little or too much	Too much sun
Foods (name)	Medicine (name)

Others	

How was the Headache relieved:

Medicines (name)

Sleep/ Rest

Others

Additional Notes

Date:...................... Day of Week:.......................

Time Occurred		Time Ended	

Type of headache you have: Tick the Right one.

Sinus   Tension   Migraine   Cluster   Hypertension

Severity on a Scale of 1-10 : Tick the right number

1	2	3	4	5	6	7	8	9	10

Triggers: Tick the Right One

Stress, anger or sadness	Loud Noises
Missed eating a meal	Period
Slept too little or too much	Too much sun
Foods (name)	Medicine (name)

Others

How was the Headache relieved:

Medicines (name)

Sleep/ Rest

Others

Additional Notes

_____

_____

_____

Date:...................... Day of Week:.......................

Time Occurred		Time Ended	

Type of headache you have: Tick the Right one.

Sinus   Tension   Migraine   Cluster   Hypertension

Severity on a Scale of 1-10 : Tick the right number

1	2	3	4	5	6	7	8	9	10

Triggers: Tick the Right One

Stress, anger or sadness	Loud Noises
Missed eating a meal	Period
Slept too little or too much	Too much sun
Foods (name)	Medicine (name)
Others	

How was the Headache relieved:

Medicines (name)
Sleep/ Rest
Others

Additional Notes

Date:........................ Day of Week:........................

Time Occurred		Time Ended	

Type of headache you have: Tick the Right one.

Sinus　　Tension　　Migraine　　Cluster　　Hypertension

Severity on a Scale of 1-10 : Tick the right number

1	2	3	4	5	6	7	8	9	10

Triggers: Tick the Right One

Stress, anger or sadness	Loud Noises
Missed eating a meal	Period
Slept too little or too much	Too much sun
Foods (name)	Medicine (name)

Others

How was the Headache relieved:

Medicines (name)

Sleep/ Rest

Others

Additional Notes

_____

_____

_____

Date:....................   Day of Week:......................

Time Occurred		Time Ended	

Type of headache you have: Tick the Right one.

Sinus   Tension   Migraine   Cluster   Hypertension

Severity on a Scale of 1-10 : Tick the right number

1	2	3	4	5	6	7	8	9	10

Triggers: Tick the Right One

Stress, anger or sadness	Loud Noises
Missed eating a meal	Period
Slept too little or too much	Too much sun
Foods (name)	Medicine (name)
Others	

How was the Headache relieved:

Medicines (name)

Sleep/ Rest

Others

Additional Notes

_____

_____

_____

Date:........................   Day of Week:........................

Time Occurred		Time Ended	

Type of headache you have: Tick the Right one.

Sinus   Tension   Migraine   Cluster   Hypertension

Severity on a Scale of 1-10 : Tick the right number

1	2	3	4	5	6	7	8	9	10

Triggers: Tick the Right One

Stress, anger or sadness	Loud Noises
Missed eating a meal	Period
Slept too little or too much	Too much sun
Foods (name)	Medicine (name)

Others

How was the Headache relieved:

Medicines (name)
Sleep/ Rest
Others

Additional Notes

_____

_____

_____

_____

Date:..................... Day of Week:......................

Time Occurred		Time Ended	

Type of headache you have: Tick the Right one.

Sinus   Tension   Migraine   Cluster   Hypertension

Severity on a Scale of 1-10 : Tick the right number

1	2	3	4	5	6	7	8	9	10

Triggers: Tick the Right One

Stress, anger or sadness	Loud Noises
Missed eating a meal	Period
Slept too little or too much	Too much sun
Foods (name)	Medicine (name)
Others	

How was the Headache relieved:

Medicines (name)

Sleep/ Rest

Others

Additional Notes

Date:..................... Day of Week:.....................

| Time Occurred | | Time Ended | |

Type of headache you have: Tick the Right one.

Sinus   Tension   Migraine   Cluster   Hypertension

Severity on a Scale of 1-10 : Tick the right number

| 1 | 2 | 3 | 4 | 5 | 6 | 7 | 8 | 9 | 10 |

Triggers: Tick the Right One

Stress, anger or sadness	Loud Noises
Missed eating a meal	Period
Slept too little or too much	Too much sun
Foods (name)	Medicine (name)

Others

How was the Headache relieved:

Medicines (name)

Sleep/ Rest

Others

Additional Notes

_____

_____

_____

Date:..................... Day of Week:......................

Time Occurred		Time Ended	

Type of headache you have: Tick the Right one.

Sinus   Tension   Migraine   Cluster   Hypertension

Severity on a Scale of 1-10 : Tick the right number									
1	2	3	4	5	6	7	8	9	10

Triggers: Tick the Right One	
Stress, anger or sadness	Loud Noises
Missed eating a meal	Period
Slept too little or too much	Too much sun
Foods (name)	Medicine (name)

Others

How was the Headache relieved:

Medicines (name)

Sleep/ Rest

Others

Additional Notes

Date:........................ Day of Week:..........................

Time Occurred		Time Ended	

Type of headache you have: Tick the Right one.

Sinus   Tension   Migraine   Cluster   Hypertension

Severity on a Scale of 1-10 : Tick the right number

1	2	3	4	5	6	7	8	9	10

Triggers: Tick the Right One

Stress, anger or sadness	Loud Noises
Missed eating a meal	Period
Slept too little or too much	Too much sun
Foods (name)	Medicine (name)

Others

How was the Headache relieved:

Medicines (name)

Sleep/ Rest

Others

Additional Notes

_____

_____

_____

Date:........................   Day of Week:..........................

Time Occurred		Time Ended	

Type of headache you have: Tick the Right one.

Sinus   Tension   Migraine   Cluster   Hypertension

Severity on a Scale of 1-10 : Tick the right number

1	2	3	4	5	6	7	8	9	10

Triggers: Tick the Right One

Stress, anger or sadness	Loud Noises
Missed eating a meal	Period
Slept too little or too much	Too much sun
Foods (name)	Medicine (name)

Others

How was the Headache relieved:

Medicines (name)

Sleep/ Rest

Others

Additional Notes

_____

_____

_____

Date:..................... Day of Week:.......................

Time Occurred		Time Ended	

Type of headache you have: Tick the Right one.

Sinus   Tension   Migraine   Cluster   Hypertension

Severity on a Scale of 1-10 : Tick the right number

1	2	3	4	5	6	7	8	9	10

Triggers: Tick the Right One

Stress, anger or sadness	Loud Noises
Missed eating a meal	Period
Slept too little or too much	Too much sun
Foods (name)	Medicine (name)

Others

How was the Headache relieved:

Medicines (name)

Sleep/ Rest

Others

Additional Notes

_____

_____

_____

Date:..................... Day of Week:.......................

Time Occurred		Time Ended	

Type of headache you have: Tick the Right one.

Sinus	Tension	Migraine	Cluster	Hypertension

Severity on a Scale of 1-10 : Tick the right number

1	2	3	4	5	6	7	8	9	10

Triggers: Tick the Right One

Stress, anger or sadness	Loud Noises
Missed eating a meal	Period
Slept too little or too much	Too much sun
Foods (name)	Medicine (name)

Others

How was the Headache relieved:

Medicines (name)

Sleep/ Rest

Others

Additional Notes

Date:........................   Day of Week:........................

Time Occurred		Time Ended	

Type of headache you have: Tick the Right one.

Sinus   Tension   Migraine   Cluster   Hypertension

Severity on a Scale of 1-10 : Tick the right number

1	2	3	4	5	6	7	8	9	10

Triggers: Tick the Right One

Stress, anger or sadness	Loud Noises
Missed eating a meal	Period
Slept too little or too much	Too much sun
Foods (name)	Medicine (name)

Others

How was the Headache relieved:

Medicines (name)

Sleep/ Rest

Others

Additional Notes

_____

_____

_____

Date:...................... Day of Week:......................

Time Occurred		Time Ended	

Type of headache you have: Tick the Right one.

Sinus   Tension   Migraine   Cluster   Hypertension

Severity on a Scale of 1-10 : Tick the right number

1	2	3	4	5	6	7	8	9	10

Triggers: Tick the Right One

Stress, anger or sadness	Loud Noises
Missed eating a meal	Period
Slept too little or too much	Too much sun
Foods (name)	Medicine (name)

Others

How was the Headache relieved:

Medicines (name)

Sleep/ Rest

Others

Additional Notes

Date:..................... Day of Week:.....................

Time Occurred		Time Ended	

Type of headache you have: Tick the Right one.

Sinus   Tension   Migraine   Cluster   Hypertension

Severity on a Scale of 1-10 : Tick the right number

1	2	3	4	5	6	7	8	9	10

Triggers: Tick the Right One

Stress, anger or sadness	Loud Noises
Missed eating a meal	Period
Slept too little or too much	Too much sun
Foods (name)	Medicine (name)

Others

How was the Headache relieved:

Medicines (name)

Sleep/ Rest

Others

Additional Notes

Date:...................... Day of Week:........................

Time Occurred		Time Ended	

Type of headache you have: Tick the Right one.

Sinus   Tension   Migraine   Cluster   Hypertension

Severity on a Scale of 1-10 : Tick the right number

1	2	3	4	5	6	7	8	9	10

Triggers: Tick the Right One

Stress, anger or sadness	Loud Noises
Missed eating a meal	Period
Slept too little or too much	Too much sun
Foods (name)	Medicine (name)

Others

How was the Headache relieved:

Medicines (name)

Sleep/ Rest

Others

Additional Notes

Date:........................   Day of Week:........................

Time Occurred		Time Ended	

Type of headache you have: Tick the Right one.

Sinus   Tension   Migraine   Cluster   Hypertension

Severity on a Scale of 1-10 : Tick the right number

1	2	3	4	5	6	7	8	9	10

Triggers: Tick the Right One

Stress, anger or sadness	Loud Noises
Missed eating a meal	Period
Slept too little or too much	Too much sun
Foods (name)	Medicine (name)

Others

How was the Headache relieved:

Medicines (name)

Sleep/ Rest

Others

Additional Notes

_____

_____

_____

Date:........................   Day of Week:........................

Time Occurred		Time Ended	

Type of headache you have: Tick the Right one.

Sinus   Tension   Migraine   Cluster   Hypertension

Severity on a Scale of 1-10 : Tick the right number

1	2	3	4	5	6	7	8	9	10

Triggers: Tick the Right One

Stress, anger or sadness	Loud Noises
Missed eating a meal	Period
Slept too little or too much	Too much sun
Foods (name)	Medicine (name)

Others

How was the Headache relieved:

Medicines (name)

Sleep/ Rest

Others

Additional Notes

Date:........................   Day of Week:........................

Time Occurred		Time Ended	

Type of headache you have: Tick the Right one.

Sinus   Tension   Migraine   Cluster   Hypertension

Severity on a Scale of 1-10 : Tick the right number

1	2	3	4	5	6	7	8	9	10

Triggers: Tick the Right One

Stress, anger or sadness	Loud Noises
Missed eating a meal	Period
Slept too little or too much	Too much sun
Foods (name)	Medicine (name)

Others

How was the Headache relieved:

Medicines (name)

Sleep/ Rest

Others

Additional Notes

_____

_____

_____

Date:........................   Day of Week:........................

Time Occurred		Time Ended	

Type of headache you have: Tick the Right one.

Sinus   Tension   Migraine   Cluster   Hypertension

Severity on a Scale of 1-10 : Tick the right number

1	2	3	4	5	6	7	8	9	10

Triggers: Tick the Right One

Stress, anger or sadness	Loud Noises
Missed eating a meal	Period
Slept too little or too much	Too much sun
Foods (name)	Medicine (name)
Others	

How was the Headache relieved:

Medicines (name)

Sleep/ Rest

Others

Additional Notes

Date:...................... Day of Week:........................

Time Occurred		Time Ended	

Type of headache you have: Tick the Right one.

Sinus   Tension   Migraine   Cluster   Hypertension

Severity on a Scale of 1-10 : Tick the right number

1	2	3	4	5	6	7	8	9	10

Triggers: Tick the Right One

Stress, anger or sadness	Loud Noises
Missed eating a meal	Period
Slept too little or too much	Too much sun
Foods (name)	Medicine (name)
Others	

How was the Headache relieved:

Medicines (name)

Sleep/ Rest

Others

Additional Notes

_____

_____

_____

Date:..................... Day of Week:......................

Time Occurred		Time Ended	

Type of headache you have: Tick the Right one.

Sinus   Tension   Migraine   Cluster   Hypertension

Severity on a Scale of 1-10 : Tick the right number

1	2	3	4	5	6	7	8	9	10

Triggers: Tick the Right One

Stress, anger or sadness	Loud Noises
Missed eating a meal	Period
Slept too little or too much	Too much sun
Foods (name)	Medicine (name)
Others	

How was the Headache relieved:

Medicines (name)

Sleep/ Rest

Others

Additional Notes

Date:..................... Day of Week:.......................

Time Occurred		Time Ended	

Type of headache you have: Tick the Right one.

Sinus Tension Migraine Cluster Hypertension

Severity on a Scale of 1-10 : Tick the right number

1	2	3	4	5	6	7	8	9	10

Triggers: Tick the Right One

Stress, anger or sadness	Loud Noises
Missed eating a meal	Period
Slept too little or too much	Too much sun
Foods (name)	Medicine (name)

Others

How was the Headache relieved:

Medicines (name)

Sleep/ Rest

Others

Additional Notes

_____

_____

_____

Date:........................   Day of Week:........................

Time Occurred		Time Ended	

Type of headache you have: Tick the Right one.

Sinus   Tension   Migraine   Cluster   Hypertension

Severity on a Scale of 1-10 : Tick the right number

1	2	3	4	5	6	7	8	9	10

Triggers: Tick the Right One

Stress, anger or sadness	Loud Noises
Missed eating a meal	Period
Slept too little or too much	Too much sun
Foods (name)	Medicine (name)

Others

How was the Headache relieved:

Medicines (name)

Sleep/ Rest

Others

Additional Notes

Date:........................ Day of Week:..........................

Time Occurred		Time Ended	

Type of headache you have: Tick the Right one.

Sinus   Tension   Migraine   Cluster   Hypertension

Severity on a Scale of 1-10 : Tick the right number

1	2	3	4	5	6	7	8	9	10

Triggers: Tick the Right One

Stress, anger or sadness	Loud Noises
Missed eating a meal	Period
Slept too little or too much	Too much sun
Foods (name)	Medicine (name)

Others

How was the Headache relieved:

Medicines (name)

Sleep/ Rest

Others

Additional Notes

_____

_____

_____

Date:..................... Day of Week:......................

Time Occurred		Time Ended	

Type of headache you have: Tick the Right one.

Sinus   Tension   Migraine   Cluster   Hypertension

Severity on a Scale of 1-10 : Tick the right number

1	2	3	4	5	6	7	8	9	10

Triggers: Tick the Right One

Stress, anger or sadness	Loud Noises
Missed eating a meal	Period
Slept too little or too much	Too much sun
Foods (name)	Medicine (name)
Others	

How was the Headache relieved:

Medicines (name)

Sleep/ Rest

Others

Additional Notes

Date:...................... Day of Week:........................

Time Occurred		Time Ended	

Type of headache you have: Tick the Right one.

Sinus   Tension   Migraine   Cluster   Hypertension

Severity on a Scale of 1-10 : Tick the right number

1	2	3	4	5	6	7	8	9	10

Triggers: Tick the Right One

Stress, anger or sadness	Loud Noises
Missed eating a meal	Period
Slept too little or too much	Too much sun
Foods (name)	Medicine (name)

Others

How was the Headache relieved:

Medicines (name)

Sleep/ Rest

Others

Additional Notes

Date:..................... Day of Week:......................

| Time Occurred | | Time Ended | |

Type of headache you have: Tick the Right one.

Sinus   Tension   Migraine   Cluster   Hypertension

Severity on a Scale of 1-10 : Tick the right number

| 1 | 2 | 3 | 4 | 5 | 6 | 7 | 8 | 9 | 10 |

Triggers: Tick the Right One

Stress, anger or sadness	Loud Noises
Missed eating a meal	Period
Slept too little or too much	Too much sun
Foods (name)	Medicine (name)
Others	

How was the Headache relieved:

Medicines (name)

Sleep/ Rest

Others

Additional Notes

_____

_____

_____

Date:........................ Day of Week:.........................

Time Occurred		Time Ended	

Type of headache you have: Tick the Right one.

Sinus   Tension   Migraine   Cluster   Hypertension

Severity on a Scale of 1-10 : Tick the right number

1	2	3	4	5	6	7	8	9	10

Triggers: Tick the Right One

Stress, anger or sadness	Loud Noises
Missed eating a meal	Period
Slept too little or too much	Too much sun
Foods (name)	Medicine (name)

Others

How was the Headache relieved:

Medicines (name)

Sleep/ Rest

Others

Additional Notes

_____

_____

_____

Date:...................... Day of Week:........................

Time Occurred		Time Ended	

Type of headache you have: Tick the Right one.

| Sinus | Tension | Migraine | Cluster | Hypertension |

Severity on a Scale of 1-10 : Tick the right number									
1	2	3	4	5	6	7	8	9	10

Triggers: Tick the Right One

Stress, anger or sadness	Loud Noises
Missed eating a meal	Period
Slept too little or too much	Too much sun
Foods (name)	Medicine (name)
Others	

How was the Headache relieved:

Medicines (name)

Sleep/ Rest

Others

Additional Notes

Date:..................... Day of Week:.....................

Time Occurred		Time Ended	

Type of headache you have: Tick the Right one.

Sinus   Tension   Migraine   Cluster   Hypertension

Severity on a Scale of 1-10 : Tick the right number

1	2	3	4	5	6	7	8	9	10

Triggers: Tick the Right One

Stress, anger or sadness	Loud Noises
Missed eating a meal	Period
Slept too little or too much	Too much sun
Foods (name)	Medicine (name)

Others	

How was the Headache relieved:

Medicines (name)

Sleep/ Rest

Others

Additional Notes

_____

_____

_____

Date:..................... Day of Week:......................

Time Occurred		Time Ended	

Type of headache you have: Tick the Right one.

Sinus   Tension   Migraine   Cluster   Hypertension

Severity on a Scale of 1-10 : Tick the right number

1	2	3	4	5	6	7	8	9	10

Triggers: Tick the Right One

Stress, anger or sadness	Loud Noises
Missed eating a meal	Period
Slept too little or too much	Too much sun
Foods (name)	Medicine (name)

Others

How was the Headache relieved:

Medicines (name)

Sleep/ Rest

Others

Additional Notes

_____

_____

_____

Date:..................... Day of Week:.......................

Time Occurred		Time Ended	

Type of headache you have: Tick the Right one.

Sinus   Tension   Migraine   Cluster   Hypertension

Severity on a Scale of 1-10 : Tick the right number

1	2	3	4	5	6	7	8	9	10

Triggers: Tick the Right One

Stress, anger or sadness	Loud Noises
Missed eating a meal	Period
Slept too little or too much	Too much sun
Foods (name)	Medicine (name)

Others

How was the Headache relieved:

Medicines (name)

Sleep/ Rest

Others

Additional Notes

_____

_____

_____

Date:....................... Day of Week:..........................

Time Occurred		Time Ended	

Type of headache you have: Tick the Right one.

Sinus   Tension   Migraine   Cluster   Hypertension

Severity on a Scale of 1-10 : Tick the right number

1	2	3	4	5	6	7	8	9	10

Triggers: Tick the Right One

Stress, anger or sadness	Loud Noises
Missed eating a meal	Period
Slept too little or too much	Too much sun
Foods (name)	Medicine (name)
Others	

How was the Headache relieved:

Medicines (name)
Sleep/ Rest
Others

Additional Notes

_____

_____

_____

Date:..................... Day of Week:.......................

Time Occurred		Time Ended	

Type of headache you have: Tick the Right one.

| Sinus | Tension | Migraine | Cluster | Hypertension |

Severity on a Scale of 1-10 : Tick the right number

1	2	3	4	5	6	7	8	9	10

Triggers: Tick the Right One

Stress, anger or sadness	Loud Noises
Missed eating a meal	Period
Slept too little or too much	Too much sun
Foods (name)	Medicine (name)

Others

How was the Headache relieved:

Medicines (name)

Sleep/ Rest

Others

Additional Notes

Date:...................... Day of Week:......................

| Time Occurred | | Time Ended | |

Type of headache you have: Tick the Right one.

Sinus   Tension   Migraine   Cluster   Hypertension

Severity on a Scale of 1-10 : Tick the right number

| 1 | 2 | 3 | 4 | 5 | 6 | 7 | 8 | 9 | 10 |

Triggers: Tick the Right One

Stress, anger or sadness	Loud Noises
Missed eating a meal	Period
Slept too little or too much	Too much sun
Foods (name)	Medicine (name)

Others

How was the Headache relieved:

Medicines (name)

Sleep/ Rest

Others

Additional Notes

Date:..................... Day of Week:.......................

Time Occurred		Time Ended	

Type of headache you have: Tick the Right one.

Sinus   Tension   Migraine   Cluster   Hypertension

Severity on a Scale of 1-10 : Tick the right number

1	2	3	4	5	6	7	8	9	10

Triggers: Tick the Right One

Stress, anger or sadness	Loud Noises
Missed eating a meal	Period
Slept too little or too much	Too much sun
Foods (name)	Medicine (name)

Others

How was the Headache relieved:

Medicines (name)

Sleep/ Rest

Others

Additional Notes

_____

_____

_____

Date:..................... Day of Week:........................

Time Occurred		Time Ended	

Type of headache you have: Tick the Right one.

Sinus   Tension   Migraine   Cluster   Hypertension

Severity on a Scale of 1-10 : Tick the right number

1	2	3	4	5	6	7	8	9	10

Triggers: Tick the Right One

Stress, anger or sadness	Loud Noises
Missed eating a meal	Period
Slept too little or too much	Too much sun
Foods (name)	Medicine (name)
Others	

How was the Headache relieved:

Medicines (name)

Sleep/ Rest

Others

Additional Notes

Date:.....................   Day of Week:........................

Time Occurred		Time Ended	

Type of headache you have: Tick the Right one.

Sinus   Tension   Migraine   Cluster   Hypertension

Severity on a Scale of 1-10 : Tick the right number

1	2	3	4	5	6	7	8	9	10

Triggers: Tick the Right One

Stress, anger or sadness	Loud Noises
Missed eating a meal	Period
Slept too little or too much	Too much sun
Foods (name)	Medicine (name)

Others

How was the Headache relieved:

Medicines (name)

Sleep/ Rest

Others

Additional Notes

_____

_____

_____

_____

Date:..................... Day of Week:......................

Time Occurred		Time Ended	

Type of headache you have: Tick the Right one.

| Sinus | Tension | Migraine | Cluster | Hypertension |

Severity on a Scale of 1-10 : Tick the right number

1	2	3	4	5	6	7	8	9	10

Triggers: Tick the Right One

Stress, anger or sadness	Loud Noises
Missed eating a meal	Period
Slept too little or too much	Too much sun
Foods (name)	Medicine (name)
Others	

How was the Headache relieved:

Medicines (name)

Sleep/ Rest

Others

Additional Notes

Date:..................... Day of Week:........................

Time Occurred		Time Ended	

Type of headache you have: Tick the Right one.

Sinus   Tension   Migraine   Cluster   Hypertension

Severity on a Scale of 1-10 : Tick the right number

1	2	3	4	5	6	7	8	9	10

Triggers: Tick the Right One

Stress, anger or sadness	Loud Noises
Missed eating a meal	Period
Slept too little or too much	Too much sun
Foods (name)	Medicine (name)

Others

How was the Headache relieved:

Medicines (name)

Sleep/ Rest

Others

Additional Notes

_____

_____

_____

Date:...................... Day of Week:.......................

Time Occurred		Time Ended	

Type of headache you have: Tick the Right one.

Sinus	Tension	Migraine	Cluster	Hypertension

Severity on a Scale of 1-10 : Tick the right number

1	2	3	4	5	6	7	8	9	10

Triggers: Tick the Right One

Stress, anger or sadness	Loud Noises
Missed eating a meal	Period
Slept too little or too much	Too much sun
Foods (name)	Medicine (name)
Others	

How was the Headache relieved:

Medicines (name)

Sleep/ Rest

Others

Additional Notes

Date:..................... Day of Week:.....................

Time Occurred		Time Ended	

Type of headache you have: Tick the Right one.

Sinus   Tension   Migraine   Cluster   Hypertension

Severity on a Scale of 1-10 : Tick the right number

1	2	3	4	5	6	7	8	9	10

Triggers: Tick the Right One

Stress, anger or sadness	Loud Noises
Missed eating a meal	Period
Slept too little or too much	Too much sun
Foods (name)	Medicine (name)

Others

How was the Headache relieved:

Medicines (name)

Sleep/ Rest

Others

Additional Notes

_____

_____

_____

Date:..................... Day of Week:......................

Time Occurred		Time Ended	

Type of headache you have: Tick the Right one.

Sinus   Tension   Migraine   Cluster   Hypertension

Severity on a Scale of 1-10 : Tick the right number

1	2	3	4	5	6	7	8	9	10

Triggers: Tick the Right One

Stress, anger or sadness	Loud Noises
Missed eating a meal	Period
Slept too little or too much	Too much sun
Foods (name)	Medicine (name)
Others	

How was the Headache relieved:

Medicines (name)

Sleep/ Rest

Others

Additional Notes

Date:...................... Day of Week:.......................

Time Occurred		Time Ended	

Type of headache you have: Tick the Right one.

| Sinus | Tension | Migraine | Cluster | Hypertension |

Severity on a Scale of 1-10 : Tick the right number

1	2	3	4	5	6	7	8	9	10

Triggers: Tick the Right One

Stress, anger or sadness	Loud Noises
Missed eating a meal	Period
Slept too little or too much	Too much sun
Foods (name)	Medicine (name)

Others

How was the Headache relieved:

Medicines (name)

Sleep/ Rest

Others

Additional Notes

_____

_____

_____

Date:........................   Day of Week:.........................

Time Occurred		Time Ended	

Type of headache you have: Tick the Right one.

Sinus   Tension   Migraine   Cluster   Hypertension

Severity on a Scale of 1-10 : Tick the right number

1	2	3	4	5	6	7	8	9	10

Triggers: Tick the Right One

Stress, anger or sadness	Loud Noises
Missed eating a meal	Period
Slept too little or too much	Too much sun
Foods (name)	Medicine (name)
Others	

How was the Headache relieved:

Medicines (name)

Sleep/ Rest

Others

Additional Notes

_____

_____

_____

Date:......................... Day of Week:.........................

Time Occurred		Time Ended	

Type of headache you have: Tick the Right one.

Sinus   Tension   Migraine   Cluster   Hypertension

Severity on a Scale of 1-10 : Tick the right number

1	2	3	4	5	6	7	8	9	10

Triggers: Tick the Right One

Stress, anger or sadness	Loud Noises
Missed eating a meal	Period
Slept too little or too much	Too much sun
Foods (name)	Medicine (name)

Others

How was the Headache relieved:

Medicines (name)

Sleep/ Rest

Others

Additional Notes

Date:........................   Day of Week:........................

Time Occurred		Time Ended	

Type of headache you have: Tick the Right one.

Sinus   Tension   Migraine   Cluster   Hypertension

Severity on a Scale of 1-10 : Tick the right number

1	2	3	4	5	6	7	8	9	10

Triggers: Tick the Right One

Stress, anger or sadness	Loud Noises
Missed eating a meal	Period
Slept too little or too much	Too much sun
Foods (name)	Medicine (name)

Others

How was the Headache relieved:

Medicines (name)

Sleep/ Rest

Others

Additional Notes

_____

_____

_____

Date:...................... Day of Week:........................

Time Occurred		Time Ended	

Type of headache you have: Tick the Right one.

Sinus   Tension   Migraine   Cluster   Hypertension

Severity on a Scale of 1-10 : Tick the right number

1	2	3	4	5	6	7	8	9	10

Triggers: Tick the Right One

Stress, anger or sadness	Loud Noises
Missed eating a meal	Period
Slept too little or too much	Too much sun
Foods (name)	Medicine (name)

Others

How was the Headache relieved:

Medicines (name)

Sleep/ Rest

Others

Additional Notes

_____

_____

_____

Date:...................... Day of Week:......................

| Time Occurred | | Time Ended | |

Type of headache you have: Tick the Right one.

Sinus   Tension   Migraine   Cluster   Hypertension

Severity on a Scale of 1-10 : Tick the right number

| 1 | 2 | 3 | 4 | 5 | 6 | 7 | 8 | 9 | 10 |

Triggers: Tick the Right One

Stress, anger or sadness	Loud Noises
Missed eating a meal	Period
Slept too little or too much	Too much sun
Foods (name)	Medicine (name)

Others

How was the Headache relieved:

Medicines (name)

Sleep/ Rest

Others

Additional Notes

Date:....................... Day of Week:........................

Time Occurred		Time Ended	

Type of headache you have: Tick the Right one.

Sinus   Tension   Migraine   Cluster   Hypertension

Severity on a Scale of 1-10 : Tick the right number

1	2	3	4	5	6	7	8	9	10

Triggers: Tick the Right One

Stress, anger or sadness	Loud Noises
Missed eating a meal	Period
Slept too little or too much	Too much sun
Foods (name)	Medicine (name)

Others

How was the Headache relieved:

Medicines (name)

Sleep/ Rest

Others

Additional Notes

Date:..................... Day of Week:.......................

| Time Occurred | | Time Ended | |

Type of headache you have: Tick the Right one.

Sinus   Tension   Migraine   Cluster   Hypertension

Severity on a Scale of 1-10 : Tick the right number

| 1 | 2 | 3 | 4 | 5 | 6 | 7 | 8 | 9 | 10 |

Triggers: Tick the Right One

Stress, anger or sadness	Loud Noises
Missed eating a meal	Period
Slept too little or too much	Too much sun
Foods (name)	Medicine (name)

Others

How was the Headache relieved:

Medicines (name)

Sleep/ Rest

Others

Additional Notes

Date:.....................   Day of Week:......................

Time Occurred		Time Ended	

Type of headache you have: Tick the Right one.

Sinus   Tension   Migraine   Cluster   Hypertension

Severity on a Scale of 1-10 : Tick the right number

1	2	3	4	5	6	7	8	9	10

Triggers: Tick the Right One

Stress, anger or sadness	Loud Noises
Missed eating a meal	Period
Slept too little or too much	Too much sun
Foods (name)	Medicine (name)

Others

How was the Headache relieved:

Medicines (name)

Sleep/ Rest

Others

Additional Notes

Date:..................... Day of Week:.....................

Time Occurred		Time Ended	

Type of headache you have: Tick the Right one.

Sinus   Tension   Migraine   Cluster   Hypertension

Severity on a Scale of 1-10 : Tick the right number

1	2	3	4	5	6	7	8	9	10

Triggers: Tick the Right One

Stress, anger or sadness	Loud Noises
Missed eating a meal	Period
Slept too little or too much	Too much sun
Foods (name)	Medicine (name)

Others

How was the Headache relieved:

Medicines (name)

Sleep/ Rest

Others

Additional Notes

Date:..................... Day of Week:.......................

Time Occurred		Time Ended	

Type of headache you have: Tick the Right one.

Sinus   Tension   Migraine   Cluster   Hypertension

Severity on a Scale of 1-10 : Tick the right number

1	2	3	4	5	6	7	8	9	10

Triggers: Tick the Right One

Stress, anger or sadness	Loud Noises
Missed eating a meal	Period
Slept too little or too much	Too much sun
Foods (name)	Medicine (name)

Others

How was the Headache relieved:

Medicines (name)

Sleep/ Rest

Others

Additional Notes

Date:........................   Day of Week:........................

Time Occurred		Time Ended	

Type of headache you have: Tick the Right one.

Sinus   Tension   Migraine   Cluster   Hypertension

Severity on a Scale of 1-10 : Tick the right number

1	2	3	4	5	6	7	8	9	10

Triggers: Tick the Right One

Stress, anger or sadness	Loud Noises
Missed eating a meal	Period
Slept too little or too much	Too much sun
Foods (name)	Medicine (name)

Others

How was the Headache relieved:

Medicines (name)

Sleep/ Rest

Others

Additional Notes

_____

_____

_____

Date:....................... Day of Week:........................

Time Occurred		Time Ended	

Type of headache you have: Tick the Right one.

Sinus   Tension   Migraine   Cluster   Hypertension

Severity on a Scale of 1-10 : Tick the right number

1	2	3	4	5	6	7	8	9	10

Triggers: Tick the Right One

Stress, anger or sadness	Loud Noises
Missed eating a meal	Period
Slept too little or too much	Too much sun
Foods (name)	Medicine (name)

Others

How was the Headache relieved:

Medicines (name)

Sleep/ Rest

Others

Additional Notes

_____

_____

_____

Date:..................... Day of Week:......................

| Time Occurred | | Time Ended | |

Type of headache you have: Tick the Right one.

Sinus   Tension   Migraine   Cluster   Hypertension

Severity on a Scale of 1-10 : Tick the right number

| 1 | 2 | 3 | 4 | 5 | 6 | 7 | 8 | 9 | 10 |

Triggers: Tick the Right One

Stress, anger or sadness	Loud Noises
Missed eating a meal	Period
Slept too little or too much	Too much sun
Foods (name)	Medicine (name)

Others

How was the Headache relieved:

Medicines (name)

Sleep/ Rest

Others

Additional Notes

Date:........................ Day of Week:........................

Time Occurred		Time Ended	

Type of headache you have: Tick the Right one.

Sinus   Tension   Migraine   Cluster   Hypertension

Severity on a Scale of 1-10 : Tick the right number

1	2	3	4	5	6	7	8	9	10

Triggers: Tick the Right One

Stress, anger or sadness	Loud Noises
Missed eating a meal	Period
Slept too little or too much	Too much sun
Foods (name)	Medicine (name)

Others

How was the Headache relieved:

Medicines (name)

Sleep/ Rest

Others

Additional Notes

Date:........................ Day of Week:........................

| Time Occurred | | Time Ended | |

Type of headache you have: Tick the Right one.

Sinus   Tension   Migraine   Cluster   Hypertension

Severity on a Scale of 1-10 : Tick the right number

| 1 | 2 | 3 | 4 | 5 | 6 | 7 | 8 | 9 | 10 |

Triggers: Tick the Right One

Stress, anger or sadness	Loud Noises
Missed eating a meal	Period
Slept too little or too much	Too much sun
Foods (name)	Medicine (name)

Others

How was the Headache relieved:

Medicines (name)

Sleep/ Rest

Others

Additional Notes

Date:..................... Day of Week:.......................

Time Occurred		Time Ended	

Type of headache you have: Tick the Right one.

Sinus   Tension   Migraine   Cluster   Hypertension

Severity on a Scale of 1-10 : Tick the right number

1	2	3	4	5	6	7	8	9	10

Triggers: Tick the Right One

Stress, anger or sadness	Loud Noises
Missed eating a meal	Period
Slept too little or too much	Too much sun
Foods (name)	Medicine (name)

Others

How was the Headache relieved:

Medicines (name)

Sleep/ Rest

Others

Additional Notes

Date:........................ Day of Week:..........................

Time Occurred		Time Ended	

Type of headache you have: Tick the Right one.

Sinus   Tension   Migraine   Cluster   Hypertension

Severity on a Scale of 1-10 : Tick the right number

1	2	3	4	5	6	7	8	9	10

Triggers: Tick the Right One

Stress, anger or sadness	Loud Noises
Missed eating a meal	Period
Slept too little or too much	Too much sun
Foods (name)	Medicine (name)

Others

How was the Headache relieved:

Medicines (name)

Sleep/ Rest

Others

Additional Notes

Date:........................   Day of Week:........................

Time Occurred		Time Ended	

Type of headache you have: Tick the Right one.

Sinus   Tension   Migraine   Cluster   Hypertension

Severity on a Scale of 1-10 : Tick the right number

1	2	3	4	5	6	7	8	9	10

Triggers: Tick the Right One

Stress, anger or sadness	Loud Noises
Missed eating a meal	Period
Slept too little or too much	Too much sun
Foods (name)	Medicine (name)

Others

How was the Headache relieved:

Medicines (name)

Sleep/ Rest

Others

Additional Notes

Date:....................... Day of Week:........................

Time Occurred		Time Ended	

Type of headache you have: Tick the Right one.

Sinus	Tension	Migraine	Cluster	Hypertension

Severity on a Scale of 1-10 : Tick the right number

1	2	3	4	5	6	7	8	9	10

Triggers: Tick the Right One

Stress, anger or sadness	Loud Noises
Missed eating a meal	Period
Slept too little or too much	Too much sun
Foods (name)	Medicine (name)

Others

How was the Headache relieved:

Medicines (name)

Sleep/ Rest

Others

Additional Notes

Date:.................... Day of Week:.......................

Time Occurred		Time Ended	

Type of headache you have: Tick the Right one.

Sinus   Tension   Migraine   Cluster   Hypertension

Severity on a Scale of 1-10 : Tick the right number

1	2	3	4	5	6	7	8	9	10

Triggers: Tick the Right One

Stress, anger or sadness	Loud Noises
Missed eating a meal	Period
Slept too little or too much	Too much sun
Foods (name)	Medicine (name)

Others

How was the Headache relieved:

Medicines (name)

Sleep/ Rest

Others

Additional Notes

_____

_____

_____

Date:....................... Day of Week:........................

Time Occurred		Time Ended	

Type of headache you have: Tick the Right one.

Sinus   Tension   Migraine   Cluster   Hypertension

Severity on a Scale of 1-10 : Tick the right number

1	2	3	4	5	6	7	8	9	10

Triggers: Tick the Right One

Stress, anger or sadness	Loud Noises
Missed eating a meal	Period
Slept too little or too much	Too much sun
Foods (name)	Medicine (name)

Others

How was the Headache relieved:

Medicines (name)

Sleep/ Rest

Others

Additional Notes

Date:...................... Day of Week:........................

Time Occurred		Time Ended	

Type of headache you have: Tick the Right one.

Sinus   Tension   Migraine   Cluster   Hypertension

Severity on a Scale of 1-10 : Tick the right number

1	2	3	4	5	6	7	8	9	10

Triggers: Tick the Right One

Stress, anger or sadness	Loud Noises
Missed eating a meal	Period
Slept too little or too much	Too much sun
Foods (name)	Medicine (name)

Others

How was the Headache relieved:

Medicines (name)

Sleep/ Rest

Others

Additional Notes

_____

_____

_____

Date:...................... Day of Week:.......................

Time Occurred		Time Ended	

Type of headache you have: Tick the Right one.

Sinus   Tension   Migraine   Cluster   Hypertension

Severity on a Scale of 1-10 : Tick the right number

1	2	3	4	5	6	7	8	9	10

Triggers: Tick the Right One

Stress, anger or sadness	Loud Noises
Missed eating a meal	Period
Slept too little or too much	Too much sun
Foods (name)	Medicine (name)

Others

How was the Headache relieved:

Medicines (name)

Sleep/ Rest

Others

Additional Notes

Date:........................ Day of Week:........................

Time Occurred		Time Ended	

Type of headache you have: Tick the Right one.

Sinus   Tension   Migraine   Cluster   Hypertension

Severity on a Scale of 1-10 : Tick the right number

1	2	3	4	5	6	7	8	9	10

Triggers: Tick the Right One

Stress, anger or sadness	Loud Noises
Missed eating a meal	Period
Slept too little or too much	Too much sun
Foods (name)	Medicine (name)

Others

How was the Headache relieved:

Medicines (name)

Sleep/ Rest

Others

Additional Notes

_____

_____

_____

Date:...................... Day of Week:......................

Time Occurred		Time Ended	

Type of headache you have: Tick the Right one.

Sinus   Tension   Migraine   Cluster   Hypertension

Severity on a Scale of 1-10 : Tick the right number

1	2	3	4	5	6	7	8	9	10

Triggers: Tick the Right One

Stress, anger or sadness	Loud Noises
Missed eating a meal	Period
Slept too little or too much	Too much sun
Foods (name)	Medicine (name)

Others

How was the Headache relieved:

Medicines (name)

Sleep/ Rest

Others

Additional Notes

Date:...................... Day of Week:........................

Time Occurred		Time Ended	

Type of headache you have: Tick the Right one.

Sinus   Tension   Migraine   Cluster   Hypertension

Severity on a Scale of 1-10 : Tick the right number

1	2	3	4	5	6	7	8	9	10

Triggers: Tick the Right One

Stress, anger or sadness	Loud Noises
Missed eating a meal	Period
Slept too little or too much	Too much sun
Foods (name)	Medicine (name)

Others

How was the Headache relieved:

Medicines (name)

Sleep/ Rest

Others

Additional Notes

_____

_____

_____

Date:..................... Day of Week:.....................

Time Occurred		Time Ended	

Type of headache you have: Tick the Right one.

Sinus   Tension   Migraine   Cluster   Hypertension

Severity on a Scale of 1-10 : Tick the right number

1	2	3	4	5	6	7	8	9	10

Triggers: Tick the Right One

Stress, anger or sadness	Loud Noises
Missed eating a meal	Period
Slept too little or too much	Too much sun
Foods (name)	Medicine (name)

Others

How was the Headache relieved:

Medicines (name)

Sleep/ Rest

Others

Additional Notes

_____

_____

_____

Date:.....................   Day of Week:.......................

Time Occurred		Time Ended	

Type of headache you have: Tick the Right one.

Sinus   Tension   Migraine   Cluster   Hypertension

Severity on a Scale of 1-10 : Tick the right number

1	2	3	4	5	6	7	8	9	10

Triggers: Tick the Right One

Stress, anger or sadness	Loud Noises
Missed eating a meal	Period
Slept too little or too much	Too much sun
Foods (name)	Medicine (name)

Others

How was the Headache relieved:

Medicines (name)

Sleep/ Rest

Others

Additional Notes

_____

_____

_____

Date:..................... Day of Week:.....................

Time Occurred		Time Ended	

Type of headache you have: Tick the Right one.

Sinus   Tension   Migraine   Cluster   Hypertension

Severity on a Scale of 1-10 : Tick the right number

1	2	3	4	5	6	7	8	9	10

Triggers: Tick the Right One

Stress, anger or sadness	Loud Noises
Missed eating a meal	Period
Slept too little or too much	Too much sun
Foods (name)	Medicine (name)

Others

How was the Headache relieved:

Medicines (name)

Sleep/ Rest

Others

Additional Notes

_____

_____

_____

Date:..................... Day of Week:.......................

Time Occurred		Time Ended	

Type of headache you have: Tick the Right one.

Sinus   Tension   Migraine   Cluster   Hypertension

Severity on a Scale of 1-10 : Tick the right number

1	2	3	4	5	6	7	8	9	10

Triggers: Tick the Right One

Stress, anger or sadness	Loud Noises
Missed eating a meal	Period
Slept too little or too much	Too much sun
Foods (name)	Medicine (name)

Others

How was the Headache relieved:

Medicines (name)

Sleep/ Rest

Others

Additional Notes

Date:.....................   Day of Week:......................

Time Occurred		Time Ended	

Type of headache you have: Tick the Right one.

Sinus   Tension   Migraine   Cluster   Hypertension

Severity on a Scale of 1-10 : Tick the right number

1	2	3	4	5	6	7	8	9	10

Triggers: Tick the Right One

Stress, anger or sadness	Loud Noises
Missed eating a meal	Period
Slept too little or too much	Too much sun
Foods (name)	Medicine (name)
Others	

How was the Headache relieved:

Medicines (name)

Sleep/ Rest

Others

Additional Notes

_____

_____

_____

Date:........................   Day of Week:........................

Time Occurred		Time Ended	

Type of headache you have: Tick the Right one.

Sinus   Tension   Migraine   Cluster   Hypertension

Severity on a Scale of 1-10 : Tick the right number

1	2	3	4	5	6	7	8	9	10

Triggers: Tick the Right One

Stress, anger or sadness	Loud Noises
Missed eating a meal	Period
Slept too little or too much	Too much sun
Foods (name)	Medicine (name)

Others

How was the Headache relieved:

Medicines (name)

Sleep/ Rest

Others

Additional Notes

Date:........................ Day of Week:........................

| Time Occurred | | Time Ended | |

Type of headache you have: Tick the Right one.

Sinus   Tension   Migraine   Cluster   Hypertension

Severity on a Scale of 1-10 : Tick the right number

| 1 | 2 | 3 | 4 | 5 | 6 | 7 | 8 | 9 | 10 |

Triggers: Tick the Right One

Stress, anger or sadness	Loud Noises
Missed eating a meal	Period
Slept too little or too much	Too much sun
Foods (name)	Medicine (name)

Others

How was the Headache relieved:

Medicines (name)

Sleep/ Rest

Others

Additional Notes

Date:.....................   Day of Week:.......................

Time Occurred		Time Ended	

Type of headache you have: Tick the Right one.

Sinus   Tension   Migraine   Cluster   Hypertension

Severity on a Scale of 1-10 : Tick the right number

1	2	3	4	5	6	7	8	9	10

Triggers: Tick the Right One

Stress, anger or sadness	Loud Noises
Missed eating a meal	Period
Slept too little or too much	Too much sun
Foods (name)	Medicine (name)

Others

How was the Headache relieved:

Medicines (name)

Sleep/ Rest

Others

Additional Notes

_____

_____

_____

Date:........................   Day of Week:........................

Time Occurred		Time Ended	

Type of headache you have: Tick the Right one.

Sinus   Tension   Migraine   Cluster   Hypertension

Severity on a Scale of 1-10 : Tick the right number

1	2	3	4	5	6	7	8	9	10

Triggers: Tick the Right One

Stress, anger or sadness	Loud Noises
Missed eating a meal	Period
Slept too little or too much	Too much sun
Foods (name)	Medicine (name)

Others

How was the Headache relieved:

Medicines (name)

Sleep/ Rest

Others

Additional Notes

Date:......................   Day of Week:........................

Time Occurred		Time Ended	

Type of headache you have: Tick the Right one.

Sinus   Tension   Migraine   Cluster   Hypertension

Severity on a Scale of 1-10 : Tick the right number

1	2	3	4	5	6	7	8	9	10

Triggers: Tick the Right One

Stress, anger or sadness	Loud Noises
Missed eating a meal	Period
Slept too little or too much	Too much sun
Foods (name)	Medicine (name)

Others

How was the Headache relieved:

Medicines (name)

Sleep/ Rest

Others

Additional Notes

_____

_____

_____

Date:........................   Day of Week:.........................

Time Occurred		Time Ended	

Type of headache you have: Tick the Right one.

Sinus	Tension	Migraine	Cluster	Hypertension

Severity on a Scale of 1-10 : Tick the right number

1	2	3	4	5	6	7	8	9	10

Triggers: Tick the Right One

Stress, anger or sadness	Loud Noises
Missed eating a meal	Period
Slept too little or too much	Too much sun
Foods (name)	Medicine (name)
Others	

How was the Headache relieved:

Medicines (name)
Sleep/ Rest
Others

Additional Notes

_____

_____

_____

Date:........................ Day of Week:........................

Time Occurred		Time Ended	

Type of headache you have: Tick the Right one.

Sinus   Tension   Migraine   Cluster   Hypertension

Severity on a Scale of 1-10 : Tick the right number

1	2	3	4	5	6	7	8	9	10

Triggers: Tick the Right One

Stress, anger or sadness	Loud Noises
Missed eating a meal	Period
Slept too little or too much	Too much sun
Foods (name)	Medicine (name)

Others

How was the Headache relieved:

Medicines (name)

Sleep/ Rest

Others

Additional Notes

Date:..................... Day of Week:.....................

Time Occurred		Time Ended	

Type of headache you have: Tick the Right one.

Sinus Tension Migraine Cluster Hypertension

Severity on a Scale of 1-10 : Tick the right number

1	2	3	4	5	6	7	8	9	10

Triggers: Tick the Right One

Stress, anger or sadness	Loud Noises
Missed eating a meal	Period
Slept too little or too much	Too much sun
Foods (name)	Medicine (name)
Others	

How was the Headache relieved:

Medicines (name)

Sleep/ Rest

Others

Additional Notes

Date:...................... Day of Week:.........................

Time Occurred		Time Ended	

Type of headache you have: Tick the Right one.

| Sinus | Tension | Migraine | Cluster | Hypertension |

Severity on a Scale of 1-10 : Tick the right number

1	2	3	4	5	6	7	8	9	10

Triggers: Tick the Right One

Stress, anger or sadness	Loud Noises
Missed eating a meal	Period
Slept too little or too much	Too much sun
Foods (name)	Medicine (name)

Others

How was the Headache relieved:

Medicines (name)

Sleep/ Rest

Others

Additional Notes

_____

_____

_____

Date:........................   Day of Week:........................

Time Occurred		Time Ended	

Type of headache you have: Tick the Right one.

Sinus   Tension   Migraine   Cluster   Hypertension

Severity on a Scale of 1-10 : Tick the right number

1	2	3	4	5	6	7	8	9	10

Triggers: Tick the Right One

Stress, anger or sadness	Loud Noises
Missed eating a meal	Period
Slept too little or too much	Too much sun
Foods (name)	Medicine (name)
Others	

How was the Headache relieved:

Medicines (name)

Sleep/ Rest

Others

Additional Notes

_____

_____

_____

Date:...................... Day of Week:......................

Time Occurred		Time Ended	

Type of headache you have: Tick the Right one.

Sinus   Tension   Migraine   Cluster   Hypertension

Severity on a Scale of 1-10 : Tick the right number

1	2	3	4	5	6	7	8	9	10

Triggers: Tick the Right One

Stress, anger or sadness	Loud Noises
Missed eating a meal	Period
Slept too little or too much	Too much sun
Foods (name)	Medicine (name)
Others	

How was the Headache relieved:

Medicines (name)

Sleep/ Rest

Others

Additional Notes

_____

_____

_____

Date:..................... Day of Week:.....................

Time Occurred		Time Ended	

Type of headache you have: Tick the Right one.

Sinus   Tension   Migraine   Cluster   Hypertension

Severity on a Scale of 1-10 : Tick the right number

1	2	3	4	5	6	7	8	9	10

Triggers: Tick the Right One

Stress, anger or sadness	Loud Noises
Missed eating a meal	Period
Slept too little or too much	Too much sun
Foods (name)	Medicine (name)

Others

How was the Headache relieved:

Medicines (name)

Sleep/ Rest

Others

Additional Notes

Date:........................ Day of Week:..........................

Time Occurred		Time Ended	

Type of headache you have: Tick the Right one.

Sinus   Tension   Migraine   Cluster   Hypertension

Severity on a Scale of 1-10 : Tick the right number

1	2	3	4	5	6	7	8	9	10

Triggers: Tick the Right One

Stress, anger or sadness	Loud Noises
Missed eating a meal	Period
Slept too little or too much	Too much sun
Foods (name)	Medicine (name)

Others

How was the Headache relieved:

Medicines (name)

Sleep/ Rest

Others

Additional Notes

_____

_____

_____

Date:.....................   Day of Week:.......................

Time Occurred		Time Ended	

Type of headache you have: Tick the Right one.

Sinus   Tension   Migraine   Cluster   Hypertension

Severity on a Scale of 1-10 : Tick the right number

1	2	3	4	5	6	7	8	9	10

Triggers: Tick the Right One

Stress, anger or sadness	Loud Noises
Missed eating a meal	Period
Slept too little or too much	Too much sun
Foods (name)	Medicine (name)
Others	

How was the Headache relieved:

Medicines (name)

Sleep/ Rest

Others

Additional Notes

_____

_____

_____

Date:..................... Day of Week:.....................

Time Occurred		Time Ended	

Type of headache you have: Tick the Right one.

Sinus   Tension   Migraine   Cluster   Hypertension

Severity on a Scale of 1-10 : Tick the right number

1	2	3	4	5	6	7	8	9	10

Triggers: Tick the Right One

Stress, anger or sadness	Loud Noises
Missed eating a meal	Period
Slept too little or too much	Too much sun
Foods (name)	Medicine (name)

Others

How was the Headache relieved:

Medicines (name)

Sleep/ Rest

Others

Additional Notes

Date:..................... Day of Week:.......................

Time Occurred		Time Ended	

Type of headache you have: Tick the Right one.

Sinus   Tension   Migraine   Cluster   Hypertension

Severity on a Scale of 1-10 : Tick the right number

1	2	3	4	5	6	7	8	9	10

Triggers: Tick the Right One

Stress, anger or sadness	Loud Noises
Missed eating a meal	Period
Slept too little or too much	Too much sun
Foods (name)	Medicine (name)

Others

How was the Headache relieved:

Medicines (name)

Sleep/ Rest

Others

Additional Notes

_____

_____

_____

Date:...................... Day of Week:........................

Time Occurred		Time Ended	

Type of headache you have: Tick the Right one.

Sinus   Tension   Migraine   Cluster   Hypertension

Severity on a Scale of 1-10 : Tick the right number

1	2	3	4	5	6	7	8	9	10

Triggers: Tick the Right One

Stress, anger or sadness	Loud Noises
Missed eating a meal	Period
Slept too little or too much	Too much sun
Foods (name)	Medicine (name)

Others

How was the Headache relieved:

Medicines (name)

Sleep/ Rest

Others

Additional Notes

Date:..................... Day of Week:.........................

Time Occurred		Time Ended	

Type of headache you have: Tick the Right one.

Sinus   Tension   Migraine   Cluster   Hypertension

Severity on a Scale of 1-10 : Tick the right number

1	2	3	4	5	6	7	8	9	10

Triggers: Tick the Right One

Stress, anger or sadness	Loud Noises
Missed eating a meal	Period
Slept too little or too much	Too much sun
Foods (name)	Medicine (name)

Others

How was the Headache relieved:

Medicines (name)
Sleep/ Rest
Others

Additional Notes

_____

_____

_____

Made in the USA
Lexington, KY
28 August 2019